breath

the essence of yoga

T0127352

breath

the essence of yoga

a guide to inner stillness

sandra sabatini

jan heron editor

chloë fremantle illustrator

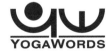

YOGAWORDS

Breath: the essence of yoga

First published by Thorsons 2000
This edition published by YogaWords, an imprint of Pinter & Martin Ltd, 2007
reprinted 2011, 2012, 2016, 2020

A catalogue record for this book
is available from the British Library

ISBN 978-1-905177-09-7

Printed by Hussar

Illustrations by Chloë Fremantle

YogaWords, an imprint of Pinter & Martin Limited
6 Effra Parade
London
SW2 1PS

www.pinterandmartin.com

a dedication

to vanda

Thanks to all my students and friends.

Sandra Sabatini was born in Australia to Italian parents, grew up in Africa, and returned to Italy in her 20s. She started studying yoga in her early 30s, and in 1985 became a pupil of Vanda Scaravelli, author of *Awakening the Spine*.

Scaravelli died in 1999 at the age of 91. She and Sandra have trained many teachers and students all over the world in a gentle but radical yoga that emphasises working with the breath, gravity and the spine.

contents

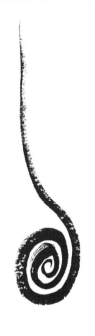

preface

Learning is fascinating. The process may start with a vague, confused need for a change. Or there will be a sudden opening for novelties – new approaches, new ways – in the usual pattern of life.

When I joined my first yoga lesson in 1975, I just felt immense gratitude for being introduced to such a vast field of ancient wisdom.

Later my body became interested in the numerous and challenging positions. Every day it was trained to perform different postures – the practice was rigorously divided into morning and evening sessions. Breathing was carried out according to strict rules and rigid timings. But at that stage it was reassuring to have a teacher and to be told exactly what to do.

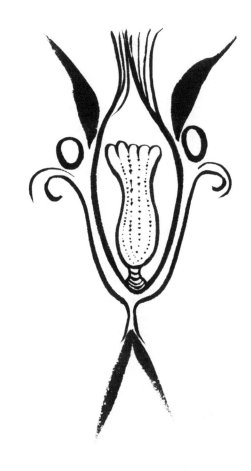

Then the birth of Chiara and three years later of Michele
brought a very different insight to my daily practice.
During labour I observed an unknown intelligence at work.
The more passive, soft and elastic I became, the more power-
fully this physical cleverness acted.

Whenever I was able to be alert but not involved,
this natural wisdom freely came into play.
Just a glimpse and the experience took me to a different state
where **listening** and **observing** became essential.
All of a sudden, my body refused to bend forward and arch
backwards: it did not want to be told what to do.
I wished only to be re-connected to that gentle, weightless
brightness I had observed at work during the birth of my
children – a primal energy that took me by the hand.

What I had learned up to that moment felt useless – my whole
being was covered by a crust of impositions. I was in a cage,
imprisoned.

But how could I possibly reverse the process? How could I start
to **unlearn**?

I needed a very special guide, a guide with a very light touch.

The first time I went to see Vanda Scaravelli, I tried to communi-
cate my strong passion for yoga and the utter confusion I had
inside me. When the tears were over, she sent me home to rest
and sleep. Two days later she invited me back to her home for
a lesson.

I was so eager to please her, so nervous, so out of touch with myself that I was unable to respond to her teaching.

What she was offering me was so beautiful that I did not know how to accept it. She invited me to open up – like a flower – from the centre. Flowers, plants and animals never hurry and yet they grow into the most wonderful variety of forms.

To learn to let go seemed like an impossible task. Vanda's respectful approach was soothing and yet she demanded total attention.

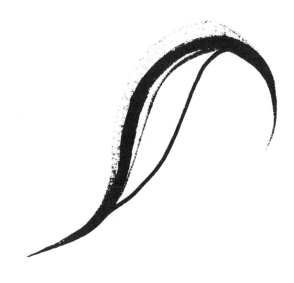

Her hands could focus for hours on the same spot until it became alive. Her words travelled straight into me; her touch gradually dispersed the crust of tensions and impositions.

And what I learned was that the breath is the key that can open thousands of doors – an infinitesimal but incredibly powerful laser capable of removing layers of encrustation.

To experience this is very often like being on the crest of an oceanic wave, a simultaneous feeling of resistance and delight.

But if fascination prevails, then opening and unravelling follows. Learning no longer comes from wanting to reach a goal or fulfil an aim, but from a gradual unfolding, an effortless blossoming.

The attention moves within to sharpen the inner eyes and the inner ears. Any subtle response is amplified. The freedom, the intelligence of the cells can float up to the surface of consciousness and there it takes you by the hand. As you learn to move with it, with the flow of it and not against it, there is immense beauty.

As the body is allowed to find its alignment between earth and sky, the practice becomes a richly rewarding voyage inwards where gifts are always offered with great generosity.

Learning is not confined to the daily practice – it leaps out into life. There is constant delight in participating and in being one with what **is:** a fusion with the object that dissolves any question and any doubt.

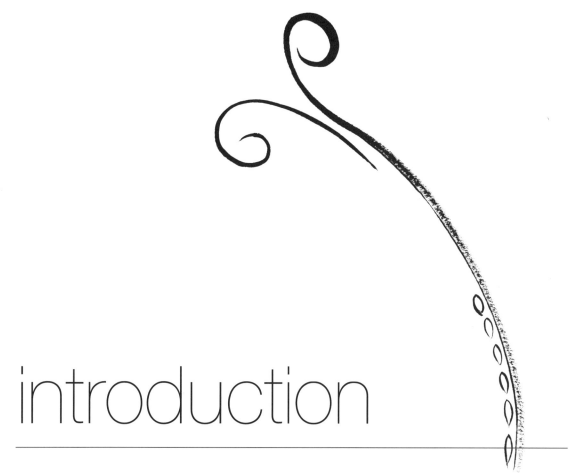

introduction

awareness of the breath and why it is so important

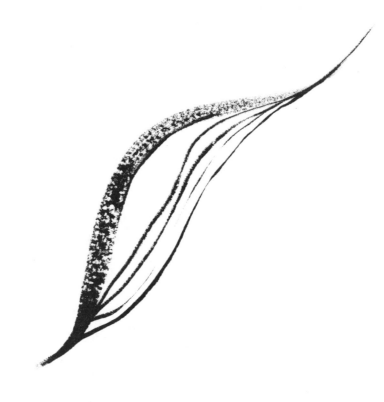

as water purifies our skin, so the breath is capable of cleaning our whole being.

but there is a difference between a calm, conscious breath that gives lightness to the body and clarity to the mind and a short, mechanical one that cripples the body and dulls the mind.

if you listen for a few minutes to the sound made by your breath on its way out of the nostrils, and then on its way back in, you will hear that it sounds uneven, hectic and rough.

this irregular, fragmented sound is an indication of how ill at ease we are with ourselves.
weeks, months, probably years of mechanical and constricted breath has the effect of laying a thick blanket on the mind and body.

there is a feeling of deep uneasiness inside.
the body sends warning signals in the shape of headaches and insomnia. we may become nervous and restless as the uneasiness increases.
concentration becomes difficult.
we start looking around for instant relief ... for something, anything that will quieten down the inner suffering and the physical discomfort.
we have lost touch with the breath.
we have moved so far away from ourselves that we have completely forgotten our closest friend.

learning to observe the breath

the transition from hectic, uneven breathing to a smooth, round, rhythmic one happens gradually and slowly but once the healing process begins, it takes you by the hand naturally and leads the way.

you may find that at the beginning of conscious breathing you experience great muscular resistance.
your ribcage feels tight, your neck is short and tense.
it may feel as if there is insufficient space in which to breathe, because this space is currently full of accumulated tension.
you may have to face another kind of resistance as well – a sort of heaviness, a sense of reluctance to meet the breath.
as a consequence, a great deal of anger and anxiety may surface.

and when you first attempt to observe the breath, your first impulse may be to try and change the pattern of breathing and give it a better shape.
but the breath refuses to be controlled.
it's like trying to control a volcano, a thunderstorm or an earth-quake.

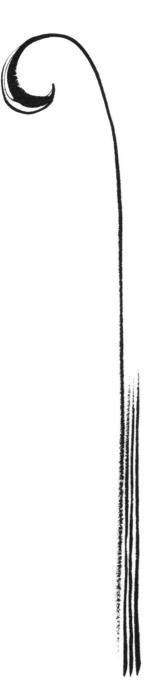

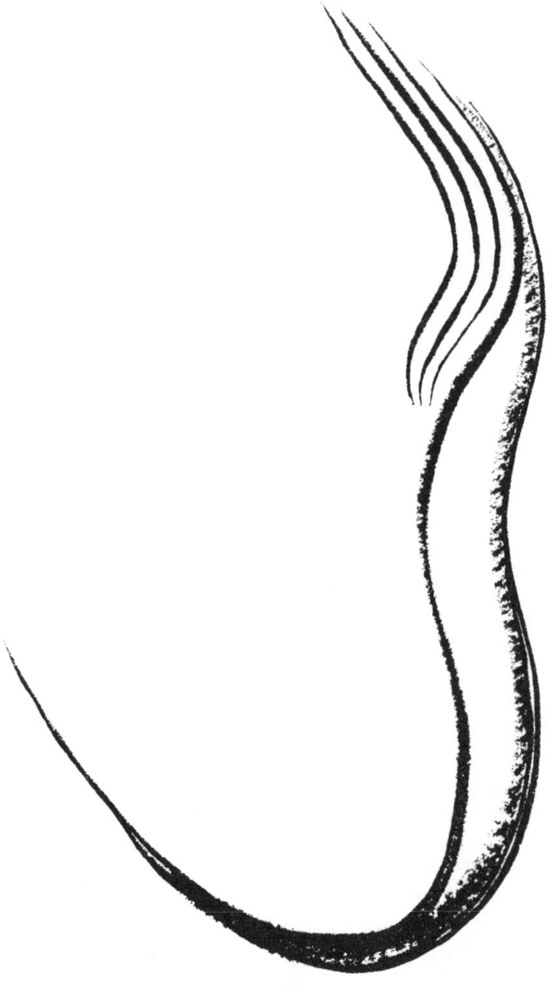

you will soon discover that there is only one way to gradually reduce the amount of poison that has been piling up over the years.

slowly, and with great kindness and gentleness, focus attention on the breath and let the impurities be carried away by the exhalation.

very slowly these impurities will be reduced and then the body can truly be nourished by the incoming breath.

the lungs open like blossoms to receive it and vitality begins to stream freely again.

it may feel as if nothing very much has happened after practising awareness of the breath.

but be sure that a series of minute rearrangements have taken place at a very deep level and that their echoes, like a ripple, will go on resounding inside you for hours, for days.

and all the time and attention you spend on observation and awareness and obtaining emptiness in the body allows the cells to absorb the full beauty and nourishment of the new breath.

breathing becomes a magic event, delicate and exquisite.

you will find that this increasing observation of your breath opens a door to the unexpected.

this simple instrument will lead to infinite discoveries.

when you are in a difficult situation, if you are in pain, or when everything seems to fail, you can reconnect to your breath and find relief.

as you learn to be in its company all the time, you wonder how you could have forgotten about it for so long.

sandra sabatini, florence

how to begin

the images and insights in this book were distilled from transcripts of sandra sabatini's classes, recorded in 1998.

their purpose is to guide and encourage the continuous process of opening, softening and lengthening that is central to sandra's approach to yoga.

it's not about achieving a position but understanding how to travel there with the breath.

if you have never practised any kind of yoga or breathing work before, this section will help you begin.

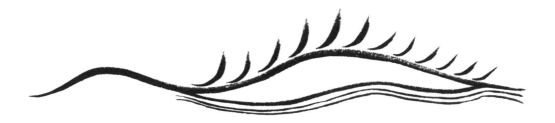

all you have to do

to benefit from the suggestions in this book
breathe
and be aware
of how you are breathing

breathe through the nostrils
easily, naturally

notice how the breath comes in and goes out
notice what happens at the end of an exhalation
notice what happens at the end of an inhalation

notice, listen, observe
by putting your attention on the breath
and just being aware

be comfortable

you can lie on your back with your knees bent
and your feet on the ground –
this is a very good position in which to begin
to observe the breath

you can also sit cross-legged, or kneel
or sit in one of the lotus positions
if you find this comfortable

take one idea at a time

take one page, one thought from the first four sections
of the book ... and use it to work with that day,
to play with, to think about or not think about

let the words float ... drift in your consciousness
don't attempt to 'do' anything
just let the words be there

this is how things happen naturally –
one step at a time, a process of gradual unfolding

it's not about doing

it's about undoing ... letting go ...
releasing ... allowing ... opening ... softening ...

as you breathe and become aware of your breath
all this will happen naturally in your body

everything will happen naturally – if you let it

the breath is **how** it happens

enjoy the benefits

as you focus attention on the breath, it becomes
very effective at cleaning and purifying at a deep level

and as the breath cleans and purifies
there is an increased feeling of lightness
and renewed energy in the body
and a greater calmness and clarity of mind.

jan heron, london

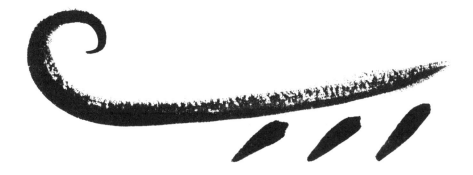

one

---

preparing the ground

at the beginning of the practice

lying on the floor
can be an encouragement to surrender
to say yes to the ground
to say yes to this process
that starts with the breathing
and leads the body
to more lightness
and in due time
more flexibility

what is essential
is quietness
inner silence
a willingness to listen

start by

lying on the ground
gently hugging the knees to the chest
the holding should not be a constant holding
as you exhale, the legs drop towards you
as you inhale, the knees move slightly away from you

allow the spine to drop into the ground
the waistline rests on the floor

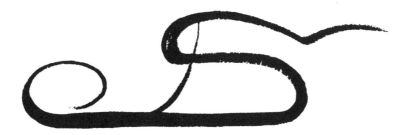

lying on your back

release the legs
and place the feet on the ground,
knees bent
arms by your side
drop the feet, drop the heels
observe the breath
and allow the spine to lengthen

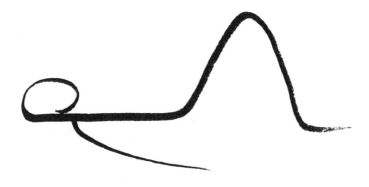

so even in a position
that looks very silent and still
there are a lot of things happening all the time

observe the spine

the spine goes up as far as the base of the head
and as far down as the tailbone

it is the whole spine that responds as a unit
to the end of the exhalation

there is a movement, a tiny tiny movement
which has to do with the rhythm of the spine
not with us wanting to go somewhere

wave

the spine acts and moves
like an organ on its own
free ... independent
with a snake-like, wave-like movement

it is the breath that creates the possibility
for the spine to move
we don't know how it moves
but it moves

surrender to gravity

gravity is your best friend
always present, always available
always ready to respond
gravity is holding you
absorbing the tension
sucking the tiredness
out of your body

relief

relief comes
from being on the ground
the ground takes care of the body
so that your attention can be
on listening to the breath

the healing ground

as you become less active
you give the ground permission
to become more active
more powerful
more healing

move inside

gather all the senses
that are usually extended towards the outer world
and turn them within
move them inside

intelligence, moving inwards

during the day
you use intelligence to catch words
to catch messages, to listen
to filter emotions

you don't need to do that now

use that intelligence, that capacity
to listen to what is taking place inside

the inner eyes

are looking at what takes place inside

the inner ears

are listening to the breath

through the breath

a constant exchange takes place
between your body and the outer world
through the breath
have a very deep respect for the breath
if the breath becomes uneven and rough
we have lost the most beautiful thing we have –
its roundness

the body loves gentleness

it is very beautiful
to follow what the body loves
the body loves gentleness

we are always so rough –
especially when it comes to movement
movement that is born with the breath
has beauty

very very simple

the minute there is a wanting
or a push or an effort
then the beauty goes away
the simplicity goes away
and it becomes something else

it's amazing
how we respond to something
very very simple
like the earth below
the warmth of hands
silence and space

distractions

when you are listening to something inside
don't be distracted by anything
everything can be an excuse
but nothing is really important
except the breath
and the lengthening of the spine
and the developing of roots –
that is really important

in time

time – in which you can observe the smallest movement within
time – in which you can see what happens

in silence
in quietness

let it happen

there is infinite time – when you look inside

reaching the centre

in yoga practice
you try to reach that centre inside your body
from which it is possible to expand ...
in yoga, with listening, with attention
with the clarity that comes from the practice
slowly slowly slowly
you touch the spot from which you can expand
into the ground and into space

reverse the process

during the day we shrink
from lack of breathing, lack of time
lack of attention, lack of love

as you get into contact with the breath
you are able to reverse this process
and obtain more space, more roots into the ground

then the body can go back to opening
lengthening, extending
in a way, you are able to change direction completely

practice is not always pleasant

there are times when you discover things
and things come undone
and there is no pain
and everything feels wonderful

and there are times when there is resistance
and when there is little understanding
of what is happening

this is natural

trying too hard

if the practice is not bringing you any joy
or discoveries or suppleness
it is because you are doing too much
trying too hard ...
and not taking time to listen

if you lose the simplicity, go for a walk

messages

when we practise, we may tell ourselves
'do this, do that'
and the entire body shrinks from these orders

instead of waiting until the body blossoms
and the breath blossoms
we are already correcting ourselves
and we do not wait for the beautiful thing
to happen naturally

the words we use to ourselves are very important
when we give ourselves negative or punitive messages
it can take a long time
to become clear again

receiving instructions from within

in our practice it is very important
how you approach everything

the attitude, the inner silence
the trust that you put in your practice –
it's like receiving instructions from within

so let these instructions travel
through the whole length of your body

healing ... opening ... and space

pay attention
but always combine it with the breath

otherwise we create limitations
it is a light attention
it never becomes heavy or serious
but it is there – always

then following the rhythm of the breath
the body is put in a situation
where there is only healing
opening and space

discover your own rhythm

trust that there is a rhythm inside you
once you discover it you are completely loyal to it
in that rhythm you find many messages of intuition and support
also there is a small voice attached –
trust this inner voice, learn to sharpen it
at one point the small voice becomes a deep voice
that is constantly there

a primal rhythm

find the key to your own rhythm
which is primal
ancient
it is there but it has been suffocated
by so much doing
and knowing

so it's like taking away layers and layers
to find this primitive rhythm
this pulse

tune in

rhythm and pattern

there is a rhythm
between attention
and undoing
attention
and letting go

there is a pattern

everyone has a different rhythm, a different pulse

release and relaxation

it's a process
it's an art

every day when you look inside yourself
and you release ...
you surrender your body to gravity
and the capacity to surrender increases
by maybe a second ...
a second and a half

feel free to yawn:

when a yawn comes up
it's only the first of millions
it's endless!
so feel free to yawn

at the end

when you want to get up from the ground
roll over to one side
and come up slowly

always roll over to one side
when getting up from a lying position

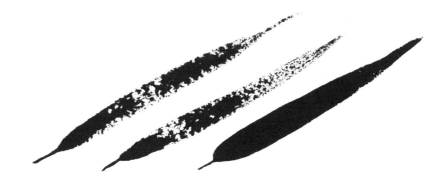

two

---

breathing: insights

breathing: how to begin

sit cross-legged or half lotus
or in full lotus or in tailor's pose
or kneel – whichever position
is most comfortable for you

make sure that the pelvis
and the legs and the knees
are really rooted to the floor

it is important to give a base to this position
so that the spine can feel free

and just breathe
through the nostrils

if you are unused to sitting there are more
detailed guidelines on pages 152 – 161

observe the breath

slowly slowly
turn all the senses that you use during the day
to perceive the outer world
inward
turn inward
to observe

you need plenty of time
in which you can peacefully observe
what happens
while the air moves out of the body
and how the air moves in
plenty of freedom
plenty of silence
so that you can observe the whole process

under a magnifying glass

observe the breath
as if it were under a magnifying glass
be interested –
as if it were something foreign, unknown
be curious
as to what happens
every time you breathe in
and breathe out
so that you can see every step

just watch
this rhythmical dance between
the external world
and the inner world
this exchange that takes place all the time

look

look at the breath
and learn how it travels
out of the body
back into space
and how it travels
from outer space
inside

listen

listening is so important
listening with the inner ear
all your attention goes to these minute movements
the minute events
that take place
while breathing

a lullaby

the breath
is round
it goes out, it comes back
it goes out, it comes back
it soothes, it heals
it is a lullaby

a breeze

the breath
is made of a very fine breeze
observe it as it travels
in and out of your body

a whispering gallery

as you sit and breathe
feel how the body becomes
a whispering gallery
where the slightest sound
is transmitted to an unusual distance –
effortlessly

round movements

when the outbreath leaves the body
the response – the answer of the body to the outbreath –
is round

it is a ripple that runs through the body

a new kind of intelligence

when you listen to the breath
you can't use the strength, the intelligence
you use during the day
you have to leave that behind

listening to the breath
requires a new kind of intelligence
it's not aggressive, it doesn't impose
it's very present
it watches
it witnesses

don't push, don't pull

allow the exhalation to travel out of the body
without leaving anything behind
only emptiness
a clean inside
don't be excited, don't be enthusiastic
just be present, in here
and let the exhalation really move,
truly move out of the lungs

the movements created by the exhalation
are so subtle
you cannot DO them
you can only accept them, receive them, welcome them ...
the rest is not in your hands
you can create a space
and then what comes in is a gift

emptiness

while exhaling ...
very slowly ...

focus your attention on
total emptiness

absorption

while inhaling ...
very slowly ...

focus your attention on
total absorption

the ripple

the exhalation travelling away from you
and the inhalation coming towards you
each create a ripple
that makes space along the muscles
that slides up and down
the entire length of your body
and opens
and lengthens

the sensation is pleasant
as you breathe in
as you breathe out
a wave goes through
the inside of the body ...
go with it

the exhalation – cleaning

the whole body responds to the outbreath
there is not one cell
not one joint
not one muscle
that is not moved by the exhalation
that is not touched
that is not cleaned

be empty at the end of the outbreath
be totally empty

the exhalation – purifying

the exhalation
is a purifying instrument
it is incredibly strong
incredibly powerful
it can create so much space
inside the body

let it travel
let the body respond to it

all the bad air

when you first start
to practise breathing
you just clean, clean, clean

expel the old air
not only the bad air of today
but all the breath that has accumulated inside –
used, but not expelled

if this burnt-out energy stays inside
it creates heaviness, dullness, blockage, resistance
if it travels out of the body
it leaves you empty
and then the new air can be really nourishing

so say yes to this exhalation
that wants to leave the body
say yes to this inhalation
that brings lightness and vitality

small black ashes

it is the exhalation that has to learn to be free
and to carry out of the body
all the unnecessary deposits
then the inhalation is just beauty, novelty
it comes, you don't have to think about it
but in the beginning
the exhalation has to be encouraged
to take away all these small black ashes
that otherwise stay inside

the exhalation is the key

keep the simplicity of this beautiful journey
of the outbreath out of the nostrils
this exhalation that creates space in between the bones
that sends you down into the ground
that sends you back up to the sky

it opens one door after another

the exhalation melts, breaks knots

the exhalation sets muscles free

the exhalation creates lightness

the exhalation creates space

where everything might happen

there is a very precise moment
in which the exhalation leaves –
gets detached from the nostrils
and that is where everything might happen

there is a sense of immense relief
a moment – one second
no more than that
when the chance
for something completely different
happens

it's only a moment

released

the end of the exhalation
is not pushed out
but released
given out
to the outer world

at the end of the exhalation
your whole being is there
waiting for the inhalation to move in

new breath

to exhale is to create space for the new breath
be empty at the end of the outbreath

this emptiness is the ground
for thousands of new possibilities ...
all we have to do is look for this total emptiness
the rest follows

tension is carried away by the exhalation
and then the body needs to settle
to find a new balance
then the new breath can come in

the new breath

observe the lungs
how gently they release the air out
no hurry ... don't push

then there is an interval
a space in which nothing happens
because the exhalation is travelling away from you
and the inhalation is travelling towards you
but it hasn't reached you yet

observe how long it takes
for the lungs to release the old air
out of thousands and thousands of pores
thousands and thousands of alveoli
and then, it's such a relief
such a beautiful moment
when everything is clean
everything is quiet ...

and the new breath comes in

passive inhalation

after the attention required by the full exhalation
become passive, porous, soft ...
be on holiday
to absorb the beauty of the in-breath

the gift of inhalation

with the inhalation
you are receiving a gift, welcoming a gift
you are absorbing
all the nourishing qualities of the air

receive the inhalation

let the inhalation
travel towards you
receive it passively

the vacuum

the outbreath creates a vacuum
and it is this vacuum
that attracts the new breath
that's why the new breath has to be passive
you don't have to think about it
it comes as a natural consequence

a song inside the body

the exhalation ...
the pause ...
the natural pause ...

the acceptance and welcome of the inhalation ...
letting the inhalation expand into you ...
the pause ...
the natural pause ...

then the exhalation ...

all these things take place on their own
and that creates a rhythm
like a song inside the body

listen to this pattern of breathing
let the breath touch the spine
move with this rhythm
which is very natural
follow it
dance with it

a special place

the pause at the end of the exhalation
and the pause at the end of the inhalation
is a special place
where nothing happens or nothing seems to happen
yet the old air is travelling away from us
and the new breath is ready to move in

in that space in between
there is silence
more than anything else
silence ... and space

learn to love the pause

learn to love the pause
give up your anxiety about the end of the exhalation
if you let go, there is more room
unexplored space
so when the new air arrives
it finds the inside of your body
very clean and shiny

explore ...

it apparently has no sound
it apparently has no movement
but at the end of the exhalation
there is a very deep purification of the cells
and by the end of the inhalation
the cells have fully absorbed the nourishment
carried in by the new breath

explore **both** pauses

there is no apprehension
there is no tightening
there is no hurry
but everything within the body becomes very very quiet

the dawn between two breaths

after the breath has entered
and just before the going out ...
bliss

after the breath has left
and just before the coming in ...
bliss

the universal pause

when the old breath has left you forever
rest
to enjoy this emptiness

when the new breath has filled you up
rest
to enjoy this fullness

the seed

the pause is the seed for meditation
you get a glimpse of what meditation is like
the space between things
between thoughts
between events

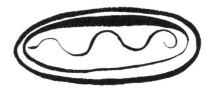

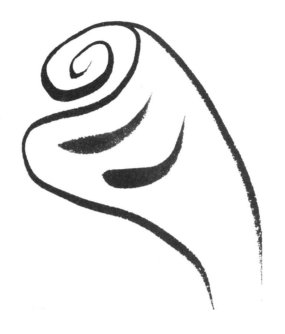

three

classic breathing

introduction

the essence of what you are doing is cleaning
the purpose of all these techniques
is to remove the 'ashes' – the impurities
that accumulate in the lungs
so that you become lighter and clearer

unfortunately these impurities are
reluctant to move out of the lungs
you do not get rid of them with strength
but by being very alert and focused
on what you are doing

how to begin

sit cross-legged or in lotus
or on a cushion or a low bench, or kneeling –
the important thing is to
be comfortable and to have your attention
focused on the breathing – not on the sitting
you can also practise all of these techniques
lying on the ground

*if you are unused to sitting you will find detailed
guidelines on pages 152 – 161*

one: kapalabhati

classical definitions:
'that which brings lightness to the skull'
dragon breath
shining skull breath

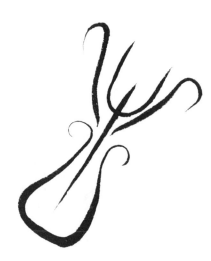

how to practise kapalabhati:

inhale and exhale normally

inhale to begin, then release the air through the
nostrils in rapid, emphatic bursts – about one per second

at the same time, the area above the pubic bone pulses –
place a hand there to feel this

after a round of 5 or 10 or 15 or more short outbreaths
and making sure the last of these is a long breath
inhale normally and exhale normally
and inhale to begin another round

practise for 5 – 10 minutes
at most

kapalabhati: guidelines

make sure any sound that is made is connected
to the exhalation – you shouldn't hear the inhalation

make sure there is no gripping inside the mouth
focus your attention
on how the muscles of the mouth
are soft, silent, loose, passive
just expel the bad air

kapalabhati carries out
the old sticky ashes from the lungs
and when they are removed
the inhalation that comes in
can really nourish
really feed the alveoli

kapalabhati: the inhalation

between rounds of outbreaths there is
this incredible inhalation
that seems to come from miles away ...

a beautiful inhalation
that travels from an enormous distance
from a very faraway place
and when it touches you
it fills up your body ... slowly, gradually

learn to be very intense and thorough
in kapalabhati
and learn also –
while waiting for the inhalation to come in
to rest deeply
deep deep rest ...
learn to drop all activities
as the body inhales ... slowly, gradually

kapalabhati: shakes

it's about rhythm
it's about releasing
cleaning
letting go
it's about exhalation
rhythmic exhalation
it's very powerful
it goes very deep inside
it really shakes the spine
and it shakes your whole being
with quick, short motions

it sets the spine free
it cleans the inside of the sinuses
it takes the dust away – the clouds

the body becomes rooted down below
and ready to absorb up above

first thing in the morning

kapalabhati takes away uncertainty – doubts
especially first thing in the morning
with the whole day in front of you
and wondering how to cope
kapalabhati can 'write the schedule' for you
in a neat, clear way

whenever you are in doubt about
how to practise, what positions to do
start with kapalabhati
it blows the cobwebs away

kapalabhati: a wonderful master

kapalabhati can be very strong
it can also be as soft as a butterfly

it teaches us a lot about the powerful qualities
of the exhalation

whenever there is a struggle in sitting
and in getting the attention
kapalabhati is a wonderful master

it's automatic, mechanical, efficient

it works for everybody

kapalabhati: even body ...

kapalabhati works on an even body

there is always one side of the body
that responds immediately
to messages that travel from the brain
through the nervous system

but there is always one side that is dull, slower –
it has more tension

because kapalabhati is a very strong muscular technique
make sure that the side that shrinks
is very firmly on the ground
and stays rooted

loose body ...

when you prastice kapalabhati
it sends the pelvis
and the legs into the ground
and at the same time
sends the spine up

you have to let this happen

if there is stiffness, tightness, rigidity
in the upper part of the body
nothing happens
so don't hold the upper part captive
let it be encouraged to loosen

kapalabhati: a very fine mixture

at one point in kapalabhati
your attention really moves inside
and you become
capable of noticing
and letting happen so many small things

you give up holding
you give up any stern attitude ...

and then something new comes up
something different
which is a mixture of respect,
lightness and silence

two: viloma

classical definitions:
'vi' denotes negation, 'loma' means hair
viloma means 'against the natural order of things'

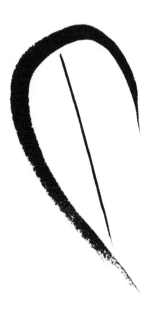

how to practise viloma:

first focus the attention on the exhalation
which is divided into two parts
inhale, and then exhale from the upper part
of the lungs
then pause ...
then exhale from the lower part of the lungs

repeat this for a few minutes

then reverse the process

inhale into the lower part of the lungs
then pause ...
then inhale into the upper part of the lungs
and then exhale

repeat this for a few minutes

then breathe normally

viloma: guidelines

exhalation:

when the attention is focused on the exhalation

the first part of the outbreath
carries all the impurities out
from the upper part of the lungs

then there is a pause – an interval – an interlude
in which the purification goes on at a deeper level

then there is another exhalation
which cleans deeply
down to the very low pit of the lungs

inhalation:

and then let the inhalation move in
accept it ... welcome it

viloma: guidelines

when the attention
is focused on the inhalation:

inhalation:

be curious about the front wall of the lungs –
how the new air gently fills up
the front of the lungs
pause ... let the air reach the top of the lungs
right under the collar bone ...
pause and then exhale

exhalation:

be curious about the back wall of the lungs
that extends as far as the waistline ...
feel its width and its full length

learn to go and live in the back wall
of your lungs
and then inhale

three: shitali

classical definition: the 'cooling breath'

how to practise shitali:

inhale:

breathe
with a slow movement through the tongue

curl up the tongue – use it like a straw
but instead of sucking in liquid
you suck in air
and then ...

exhale:

very very very slowly
through the lips
like blowing out a candle
but without extinguishing the flame

slowly slowly slowly
you let the chin drop towards the chest
the movements are always round
without interruption

shitali: guidelines

when you inhale
and absorb the air through the tongue
it's a gentle constant smooth movement

when you exhale
and release the air out
it's like drops falling out of your mouth
very very very softly

the more you relax the shoulders
the more you leave them empty and passive
the better the head is going to move
roll the chin towards the ceiling
and then slowly slowly slowly down

four: mumbling breath

classical definition:
bhramari pranayama means 'big black bee'

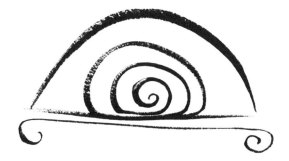

how to practise the mumbling breath:

it can be practised sitting or standing
or lying on your back with your feet on the floor
at any time of the day

mumbling breath while sitting

inhale through the nostrils
and then exhale through almost closed lips
and make a mumbling, buzzing sound like a bumblebee

the sound travels through trembling lips
and a cleansing, purification takes place
along the spine

this mumbling exhalation is cleaning
the inside of the body
with vibrations, with sounds

the slightest sound is carried
to the furthest periphery of your being

mumbling breath while standing

as the mumbling breath moves out of the lips
let the whole body respond to it
at the very very end of the mumbling breath
the heels are extended, are lengthened,
are released into the ground

encourage the centre of the foot to blossom
and encourage the centre of the hands to blossom
just a reminder –
so that this echo reaches the hands
and reaches the feet

it's not 'doing'
but deep listening, letting it happen,
a thorough respect

mumbling breath while lying with feet on the floor

as the mumbling breath moves out of the lips
the whole spine lengthens
the pelvis drops to the ground
the shoulders release and rest on the floor

there will be deeper roots
under your feet
and more space and lightness
in the shoulders
at the end of the practice

at the end

after practising any of these exercises
leave space for a few minutes of
simple breathing

then rest lying on the ground
for at least a few minutes
perhaps covered with a blanket
as the body cools down

these breathing techniques are powerful
things are shaken and stirred and moved
and you need time to assimilate any changes
that have occurred
and to rest

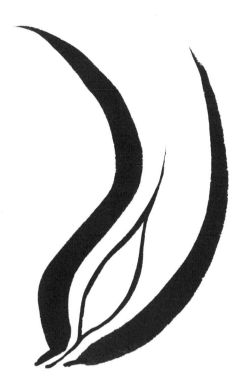

four

images

introduction

these are visual ideas to help
you while breathing ... sitting ... standing –
symbols to work with, to play with
suggested by the natural movements of the breath
in the body, and from the natural world
with which you connect while practising

the tip of the nose

when you are breathing quietly
you need to focus your attention somewhere
choose to pay attention to the tip of the nose
the air moves out of the nostrils
it touches the tip of the nose
when it comes back, before entering
it also touches the tip of the nose

observe the gentle sound of the breath as it moves out
and touches the tip of the nose
and the gentle sound of the breath as it moves in
from space and touches the tip of the nose

roots and wings

when standing
the spine moves and extends
between the ground below
and the sky above
and the body fits into this dimension
where the feet can develop roots
where the spine can dance
and where the arms one day can turn into wings

flying

while the legs and the pelvis belong to the ground
and respond to gravity
the arms like to fly
so do not hold them tight

they can then expand away from the spine
and open into space

gently – let them attempt to fly

the lightness ... the freedom
the capacity to expand
to fly ...
all the action first takes place
from the waist down
then the upper part follows
and the arms feel like wings

the spiral

the habit of thinking only
of horizontal and vertical movements
often prevents us from experiencing
the spiral one

spiral movements
are **longer in time**
and **wider in space**
than vertical and horizontal ones
applied to the breath

this is an image to employ while breathing
it facilitates the exit and entrance of air

let the old breath travel out of the body
in a spiral unwinding movement
the spiral moves around the spine
in front of the spine
and around the back of the spine
so that the journey of the breath
out of the body becomes longer
find your own rhythm
and let this unwinding spiral movement end
where the tailbone is

release – and enjoy the travelling in of the new breath

rain of light

after the emptiness of the outbreath
let your body be filled up by vital essence
to the top of the head ... and beyond ...

until it tumbles over the sides
and falls down
like a rain of light

the ripple

as the exhalation moves out of the body
and as the inhalation moves into the body
the whole of the body
is touched by a ripple
and all the stiffness, the holding, the thinking
goes away

go with it
go with the flow
this beautiful inner movement – the ripple
that the body loves so much

vortex

as you breathe
as the air goes out
it creates a wide vortex
that carries out stagnant sediment

the air that comes in
follows the same path
and brings in
fresh new particles

fireworks

when the outbreath has burned all the impurities
wait ... wait ... wait ...

then the inhalation is like fireworks
with sparkles, thousands of sparkles
dancing in the air around you

snake charmer

the spine is not vertical
it is a snake that's dancing all the time

the breath plays the tune
and the spine dances ...

there is music that goes on all the time

the epicentre

there is a place
between the base of the spine
and the pubic bone to the front
where many muscles
and nerves meet –
like a plexus

it's the epicentre

as the exhalation moves out of the body
it creates an echo
when it reaches this place –
the epicentre

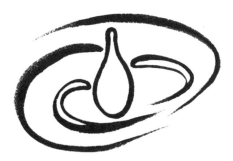

clearing the path

exhalation
is the key
with which you can enter
the roundness
the beauty of the breath

what happens to the body
during the exhalation
is like clearing the path
taking away all the weeds

like a breeze

breathe, breathe, breathe
and as you breathe
the spine can be touched and touched and touched again
until it floats
it's like a breeze running through a field of grass

waves

the body always moves in round movements
there is nothing vertical
movements are like waves
you have to go with them

each time you breathe in
and each time you breathe out
it's like offering your body to this wave
that runs up and down
up and down
the whole length of your body

the spring

at the end of the outbreath
the pelvis and legs respond
by sinking deeply into the ground

the inhalation that follows
naturally resembles
the surging up of a spring

feel nourished by it

the river

the back of the spine is like
the bed of a river
the breath is the river
you sense – at the same time –
the riverbed, the riversides
and the flowing river

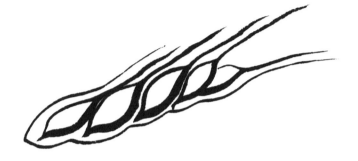

five

tiny yoga

introduction

these are guidelines and suggestions
for approaching
a few very simple yoga positions:
standing, forward bend, dog pose, cobra, tree

there are ideas to work with when you are
practising these positions –
how to move with the breath
how to create length in the spine,
and to become more grounded ...
working gently, gradually,
softly, naturally

in any yoga position: the priority

if a position does not come
or doesn't look very beautiful
nobody really cares

but if you lose the roundness of the breath
the breath becomes coarse and cross
your whole being is upset ...
so the quality of the breath remains the priority

if movement, lengthening, comes with the breath
it has roundness, grace
an easiness, a simplicity
this quality of movement is only obtainable
if it happens at the end of the exhalation

create the possibility

you have to create the possibility
for movement – lengthening, extension
to take place
create space all the time
by breathing and giving in to gravity
breathing and giving in to the earth

it doesn't come
from wanting to **do** the position
it comes from staying
being here, breathing
then something happens –
a small miracle

rigidity comes from pulling the concentration
back to the body
and making it **do** ...
instead, quiet awareness,
constant and soft
lets you watch
and be with the moment

set the spine free

all positions
are meant to create
more and more distance
between each vertebra
of the spine

so the first thing is to set the spine free
which sets the whole body free
and then you can decide
would you like to go backwards?
would you like to go forwards?
would you like to go sideways?
but the first thing is to set the spine free ...

standing

tadasana

mountain pose

how to begin:

stand with feet about hip width apart
and with the outer edge of the feet
parallel to the edge of the mat
breathe normally, quietly
allow the heels to sink into the ground
drop the shoulders
observe the breath

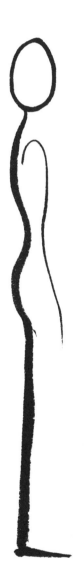

while standing: observe the breath

breathe ...
at the end of the exhalation
the heaviness of weight you sometimes find
inside the chest, the head, the arms
slowly changes location
it moves towards the pelvis
it moves to the legs
and it stays inside the pelvis
it stays inside the legs
so that the upper part of the body
becomes light, weightless

the hourglass

at the beginning of the practice
the upper part of the trunk
is too full of noises, emotions
habits, struggles

as time goes by, like the sand
in an hourglass
it all travels down
into the lower part of the body
and, through the heels
into the earth

something unexpected

at the very very end of the exhalation
something happens
some physical answer to the exhalation
and the possibility for movement in the spine
and the body
is created –
welcome the new breath

while standing: breathe with your feet

breathe with your feet
be in your feet
go and live inside your feet

and at the very end of the exhalation
dismiss the heels

it's very important
that at the end of the exhalation
the feet receive the message of spreading
so that contact with the ground
becomes more intelligent
then the roots grow stronger and thicker
into the ground
and the impulse that travels through the spine
up towards the base of the skull
encourages the opening and expansion
of the upper part of the body

while standing: unwind and lengthen

the body becomes very open, very ready
and eager to change
according to the pull that comes from underneath
and according to the attraction
that comes from the sky

slowly, slowly the perception of the body changes
activated, stimulated
by the earth below and the sky above
and the spine is able to unwind and lengthen
between these two poles

while standing: let go

as you stand and breathe
feel that you are about to fall backwards
and instead of gripping
release the toes
at that very moment

there is no need to be afraid, or grip
just release the toes
the big toe, more than anything else
and make it really long ... then rest

while standing: consider the poor toes

what happens when you move in a hurry,
when you move without combining
movement with breath
is that the body shrinks from the periphery
towards the centre, the spine
your feet suffer a great deal
from this lack of combination between
movement and breath
and the poor toes suffer tremendously
because they shrink, they curl up
they cling to the ground

so whenever you look down at your feet
and you see that they are gripping
it could be that there is something
being held somewhere ...
it could be in the mouth, the diaphragm
it could be along the spine

so just stay ... and exhale
until the message crawls to the feet
and the gripping goes away

the little toe

pay attention to the little toe
it looks so small and insignificant
but has so much to do with your balance
and the way you walk

around the foot

breathe in a circle
around the foot

circumnavigate

make a little trip
with every breath –
just breathe in and out

while standing: blossoming

in Medieval and Indian drawings
you'll see an eye in the centre of the foot
and in the centre of the hand
it's a symbol
but it is really something that physically
takes place at the end of the exhalation –
this opening

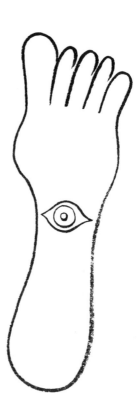

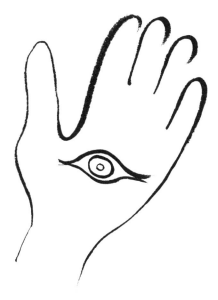

after each exhalation
there is a tiny blossoming or yawning feeling
that takes place inside the foot
and also takes place inside the hands
and you just let it happen

it's not about doing
but letting this tiny little message
travel as far as the hands
and as far as the feet

while standing: simply being

there is this contact between our feet and the ground
there is this powerful friend – gravity
that pulls our feet, our heels
back into the ground

and then there is this external ally
space – the sky
which also attracts the top of our spine

while standing: simply being

so just by simply being
by simply standing
the body is already encouraged to move
in a different dimension

at one point
the balance is just different
and you are no longer leaning forward
or leaning back
but in equal balance
between the earth
and the sky

your body is communicating
with the ground underneath
and the space up above

while standing: oscillation

there is a diagonal movement
that runs from the base of the big toe
towards the outer edge of the heel
as you stay in this position
and breathe
the feet expand and the heels drop
and there is this ripple that goes up and down the spine
all the time
at one point, the body gets into
a tiny oscillation

while standing: ask yourself ...

yes, you're touching the ground
but how?
how are you connecting to it?
how are you discharging tension into it?
how are you gathering new strength from it?

this interaction makes an incredible difference
to your wellbeing

while standing: change direction

at the end of the exhalation
the roots travel into the ground
and the upper part becomes light
in this way, we are able to completely change direction

during the day we shrink
now, instead, as we get in contact with the breath
and with the ground
we are able to reverse this process
that's caused by lack of breathing,
lack of time, lack of attention,
lack of contact with the ground
and obtain more space
more roots into the ground
and the body can go back to
opening ... lengthening ... expanding

tiny yoga

take a small step forward

the feet open ...

breathe out ...

the outer edges of the feet
gather strength
from the ground

tiny yoga

as you exhale
gently accompany the journey of the exhalation
with a slow slow slow blossoming
of the centre of the foot
and the centre of the hands

at the end, the heels are pulled
more heavily to the ground
and the wrists are attracted
to the ground as well

then take another step forward ...

forward bend

uttanasana

how to practise forward bend:

from standing, moving only at the end
of an exhalation
gradually fall forward
allowing the spine to lengthen
drop the heels
make sure the feet are really rooted to the ground
and breathe – and rest

come up slowly, moving gently with the exhalation
gradually unfurling the spine
coming back to standing position

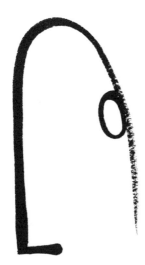

sitting positions

padmasana – half lotus
siddhasana – 'adept's pose'
baddha konasana – 'tailors pose'
simple cross legged

how to approach the sitting positions:

sitting with legs apart

bend in one leg at a time
cradling it in the arms, unwind the leg at the
hip socket

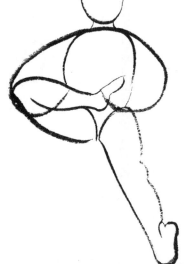

and then the other side

with the breath
open the groin
open the ankle, roll open the foot

breathing down through the pelvis
and the sitting bones
grounding the lower half so that
the upper part of the body can be free

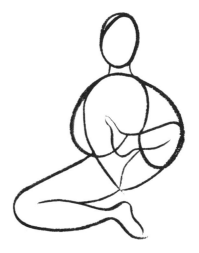

siddhasana:

place one foot on the floor
with the heel at the centre
and the other foot on the opposite calf

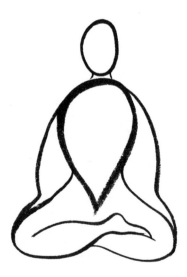

padmasana:

place the left foot on the right thigh
and the right foot on the left thigh

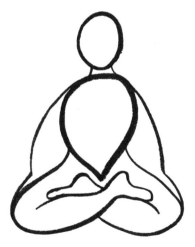

baddha konasana:

place the soles of the feet and the heels together
and allow the thighs to drop

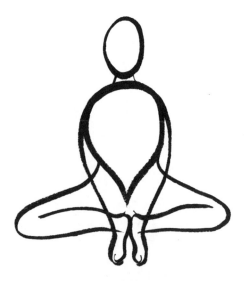

simple cross legged

simply cross the legs at the ankles

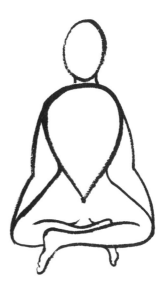

while sitting: opening with the breath

not forcing, pushing or pulling
if the knees or hips are stiff
but opening with the breath
moving at the end of the exhalation
leaning forward
letting the knees fall to the ground
and changing position of the legs frequently

while sitting, ask yourself

maybe you have been in this position
hundreds of times
but are you really unwinding ...
opening the groin
are you giving the knee the possibility to open
without pain, without pressure?
are you giving the ankle the possibility
of rolling open
and the heel to turn?
and the foot to open?

the wish to extend

in any sitting position
when the sitting bones hit the ground
the ground hits back
and creates a space along the lumbar vertebrae

then the lumbar vertebrae are able to carry
a ripple to the base of the skull
this ripple is the wish to become long
the wish to extend

this wish to extend
comes when the listening is there
and the will is gone
there is no wanting to do this or that
no trying to create this or that
not making it up

it takes place because you are breathing
everything happens between the end of the exhalation
and before the inhalation arrives ...

while sitting: the beautiful combination

nothing stays the same in the sitting positions –
or in yoga practice
there is rest, there is action ...
nothing lasts for more than a few seconds
otherwise it creates a conflict
and that's exactly what you want to get rid of

make sure all the weight is located in the pelvis
yawn ... extend ... exhale
hips get together, spine extends

and it's always this beautiful combination of
breath ... spine ... the earth ... space ...
here you are

cobra

bhujangasana

preparing for cobra

lie face down on the ground
the arms along the side of the body
feet slightly turned in
and breathe

then place the hands at the side of the body
first near the shoulders for a few breaths
and then near the ribcage, where the floating ribs are

relax the shoulders, the arms, the pelvis
drop the bones
the body becomes very long, very silent
the ground is very close
and there is a possibility for something different
something special to happen

cobra: the floating spine

lying face down
preparing for cobra
don't be surprised by a sudden movement
it's because the spine is very independent
it loves to dance
it loves to float

as you come up
let the wrists be pulled by the earth below
so that there is no tension whatever
in the shoulders
as you go down again

relax the arms down by the side
rest and give the spine another chance
another possibility
to extend even further ...

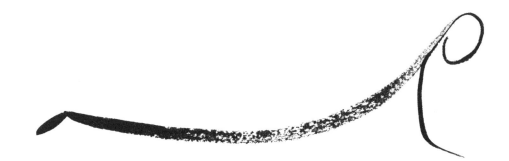

cobra: let it happen

don't move into the doing realm
breathe ... stay ... wait ... listen

observe all the ripples
encourage the roots to become deeper
heavy long earthbound legs
and then the upper part has only one possibility:
to float, to take the shape of the cobra –
its hood exposed

let the hands drop and the wrists drop
and the ground becomes more powerful, more active
and pulls the wrists down
drop the pelvis and the pubic bone into the ground
and the upper part of the body
starts floating up

cobra: following

it's about encouraging and obtaining a movement
that is whole, that spreads through the whole body
and the body is stimulated to respond as a whole

when you wait
for the exhalation to leave the body
then you can move
but without imposing on the body

just listen to the body
let the breath touch the spine
extend, and then move
you follow

you don't impose, you follow

dog pose

adhomukhasvanasana

how to practise dog pose:

begin with the knees and hands
flat on the ground
spend some time breathing, drop down through
the wrists, palms, knees, toes ...

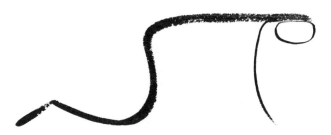

with an exhalation, let the tailbone
extend away from the shoulders
let the spine lengthen
keep the shoulders soft
breathe and lengthen

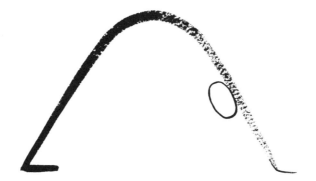

diagonal extension in dog

in dog pose
concentrate on the right hand and the left foot

open the right hand
open the left foot
and extend the spine in between
these two points

then do the opposite

there is a rhythm there
and the capacity to watch, to observe what takes place
without being overwhelmed by your body

then come back down
onto your knees
and then rest in child's pose

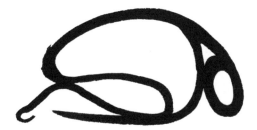

tree position

vrikshasana

how to practise tree position:

start by standing
breathing down through the feet
now allow all your weight to go down
through one side only
and when you have achieved this new balance
raise the other foot from the floor
let the pelvis drop, let the spine lengthen
and then place the foot on the thigh
of the straight leg
you can put your hands on the waist
or above your head

breath: the essence of yoga

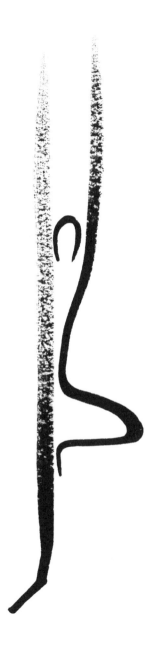

tree: insights, guidelines

this position is about equilibrium:
an effortless state
where the body is re-aligned
between earth and sky

restoring balance

observe how your feet exchange commands
with the floor –
one tends to be very active
the other very dull and passive

in the balancing position
talk firmly to the lazy foot
encourage it to open and spread
while you stimulate the outer edge of the foot
the inner arch comes back to life
and balance is restored

on your own

it is lovely to be in a group
with a teacher
someone who indicates the way in
so that the listening, the attention
becomes more alive, more vital

but the discoveries, the real miracles
happen when you are on your own

it's not a lonely journey
but one full of interaction and gifts

finally: techniques – positions

all positions are like toys
we take them and we play with them
and we leave them

the process is to be able to listen
with an alert mind
to the rhythm of the movements
but we need lots and lots of toys to play with
so that our practice doesn't become
boring, mechanical, repetitive

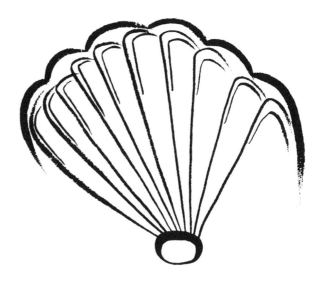

six

---

sun salutation

the sun salutation is an ancient sequence –
a prayer, a play, a dance
you can surrender to it

it isn't easy to plan your practice,
especially first thing in the morning
but you can slide into the sun salutation
without thinking ... just being aware
of the flow of the movement

if you start the day like this
with a dance or prayer
then you stimulate the dialogue between your body,
the ground and this vast light space above you

if you then sit and breathe afterwards
you have already touched the ground
and expanded into space
so your body is already in communication
with the external elements
and this continues into the breathing practice

sun salutation: the sequence

1   standing, hands in prayer position
        pay attention to how the feet touch the ground
        how they connect you to the earth

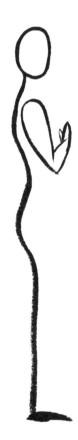

2   arms fly up, like wings
the spine extends, gently bending backwards

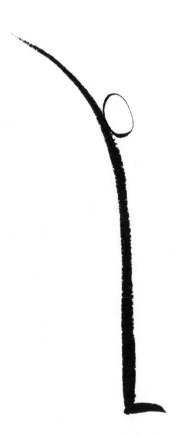

3   fall forward in forward bend
palms of the hands flat on the ground
if possible
at the end of the exhalation
there is a softening in the feet – an opening
and an opening in the hands

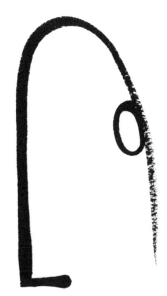

4   send the right foot back
slowly let the head rise, feeling
the ripple along the spine and then
drop the head, keeping the chin in
exposing the nape of the neck

5   send the left foot back
drop down through the wrists
flat back
the heels are encouraged to move away from the toes

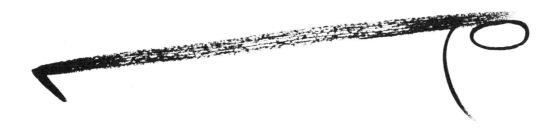

rest and breathe :

drop the knees
keeping the hands where they are
sink into child's position

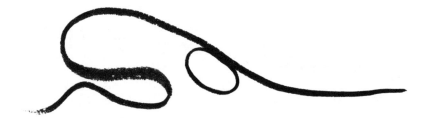

6 feeling a wave-like movement in the spine
unfurl it, scooping through the elbows

7   let the spine unfold in cobra position

8   send the tailbone back
       allow the arms and the legs to straighten
       and come into dog position

       as the breath moves out of the nostrils
       with the exhalation, the tailbone moves away from you

       breathe ... lengthen ...
       keep the shoulders very soft
       play with the spine

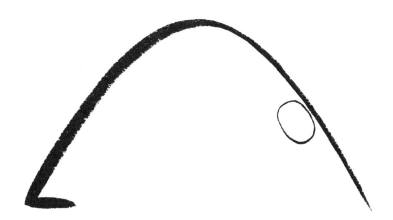

9   bring the left foot forward
and place it between the hands
slowly raise the head and drop it again,
exposing the nape of the neck

10   bring the right foot forward to join
the left, feet about hip width apart
in forward bend
keep your brain inside your feet
roots grow under your feet
and your toes are very very long

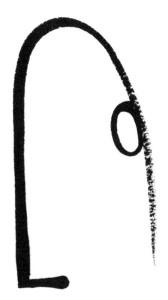

11 slowly come up into backbend position
raising arms like wings
and bringing them over the head

inhale and exhale a few times
to allow the spine to lengthen

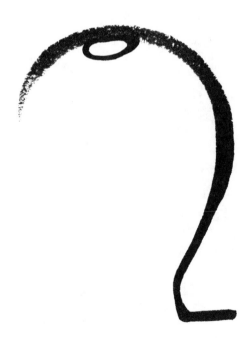

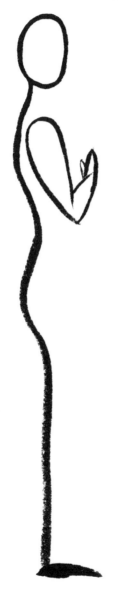

12   bring the hands back into prayer position

if the breath has become uneven, rest until it is
round and soft again

then repeat the sequence on the other side
sending the left leg back first

sun salutation: wave-like

in the beginning
you have to learn the sequence
then you can combine the positions
and make them flow
until it becomes like a wave

in each position there is a wave-like movement
the more you let yourself be carried by it
the small ones become
one big beautiful wave

sun salutation: moving with the breath

always move with the breath

it is the whole body
that responds to the exhalation
it is the whole body
that responds to the inhalation
it is the whole body
that is going to slide into movement

wait until the exhalation
with its purifying quality
creates space
creates distance
creates the possibility
for movement to take place

then breathe in

sun salutation: rhythm and waiting

wait ...
wait until each position has become quiet
grounded
as if you were meditating

let each position
become very simple
essential
innocent
clean
light
lose intentions, knots
make the body something new
in each position

sun salutation: breathe and observe

think of it as a dance
with attention to the breath
that should never become short
or uneven or gross

whenever there is a difficulty
just stay with the position
and breathe
until the position becomes round
clean
wait until the intelligence moves from the
front part of the body to the back

when you observe what happens
you acquire the necessary perspective

sun salutation: earth and sky

keep contact with the earth and the sky
the earth pulls your legs
your feet, your pelvis
the sky encourages expansion and lightness
in the upper part of the body

you're slowly pushing the body back
to a dimension where the earth works
as a very close friend
and the sky is helping by
creating this possibility for expansion ...
it's like playing with two wonderful friends

it's a dance between earth and sky

sun salutation: born to dance

the spine was born to dance

the spine dances with the breath
the spine is touched by the breath
any wanting, any aim
takes away that freedom
that chance, that possibility
for the spine to dance

think of it as long
and very very flexible

creating distance along the spine
that's what we have lost
but it can return

explore the infinite ...

the sun salutation can be an exploration
a voyage into the thousands of movements
we never really explore during the day
they are all there ...
standing, forward bends, backbends ...
and the body is encouraged,
fascinated by the opening
the growing and the grounding

in life, we set our boundaries
far too close
far too soon

in sun salutation, in yoga practice
you can go beyond your boundaries
and explore infinite possibilities

centring: while sitting

'consider your essence as light rays
rising from centre
to centre up the vertebrae
and so rises **livingness** in you'

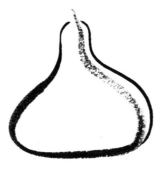

'attention between the eyebrows, let mind be before
thought. Let form fill with breath essence to the top
of the head, and there **shower as light**'

'touching eyeballs as a feather, lightness between them
opens into heart and there permeates the cosmos'

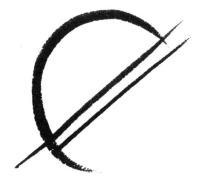

'feel your substance, bones, flesh, blood, saturated
with **cosmic essence**'

'suppose your passive form to be an empty room with walls of skin – **empty**'

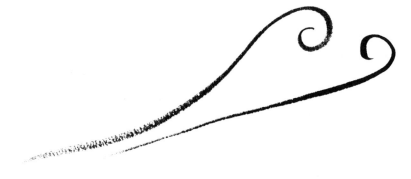

'unminding mind, keep in the middle – **until**'

'at the start of sneezing, during fright, in anxiety,
above a chasm, flying in battle, in extreme curiousity,
at the beginning of hunger, at the end of hunger,
be uninterruptedly **aware**'

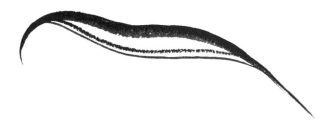

'as waves come with water and flames with fire, so
the universal waves **with us**'

these sutras, and the one quoted on page 209
are from sanskrit manuscripts
transcribed by paul reps in *Zen Flesh, Zen Bones*

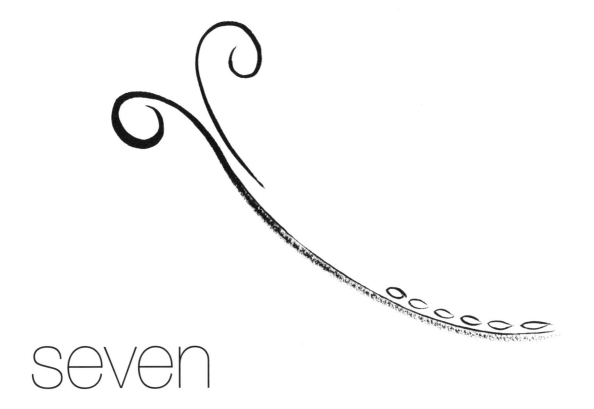

seven

---

at the end: rest

shavasana

shava means a corpse

lie on your back
with your legs bent for a few minutes
and your arms by your side
you may like to cover yourself with a blanket
let everything drop
let everything rest

then stretch out your legs in front of you
in shavasana

'place your whole attention in the nerve, delicate
as the lotus thread, in the centre of your spinal
column

in such be **transformed**'

in shavasana

in shavasana
the body gives in
surrenders the stronghold
of the mind

in shavasana
the body does not only elongate
does not only grow in length
but also in width

at the end of the practice
there is this deep wish to rest
the bones want to rest
the bones of the head
the bones of the shoulders
the arms
the bones of the pelvis
the legs

in shavasana: deep rest

as you lie on your back
let the breath float in and out
then just listen to that wish
that very strong wish
that the body has for deep rest
the bones also wish for deep rest
so in shavasana everything is going to rest
the brain, the lungs, the heart
all the internal organs
the muscles are going to rest
the bones are going to rest
the eyes are going to rest
they slide down towards the base of the skull
the skin is going to rest

everything is going to be quieter

in shavasana: release tiredness, find new strength

when the body is in contact with the ground
it can release tiredness
unload weight and tension
and tightness
because the ground is there to absorb it
to suck it out of the body

then when space is created
the ground moves in
and brings you new energy
new vitality
new strength

in shavasana: head rest

the inside of the head needs to rest
the two hemispheres of the brain
slide away from each other

there is new space between the two
and the head is able to be more silent
more quiet

this silence travels to the rest of the body
and it reaches the palms of the hands
and the soles of the feet

in shavasana: gold

at the end of the practice
lying in shavasana
the superfluous leaves the body
and disappears into the ground

only **gold** remains

from the song of mahamudra

at first, the mind tumbles
like a waterfall

in mid-course, it becomes calm
like a river flowing slowly

in the end, it is an ocean
where two halves merge in one

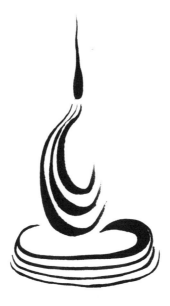

also from **YogaWords**

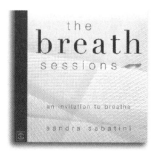

The Breath Sessions (audio CD)
an invitation to breathe

Sandra Sabatini

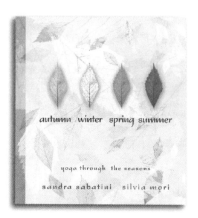

Autumn, Winter, Spring, Summer
yoga through the seasons

Sandra Sabatini and Silvia Mori

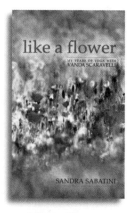

Like a Flower
my years of yoga with Vanda Scaravelli

Sandra Sabatini
photographs Dr David Darom

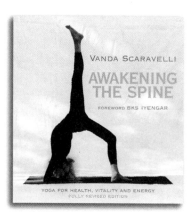

Awakening the Spine
yoga for health, vitality and energy

Vanda Scaravelli

visit **www.pinterandmartin.com**
for further information, extracts and special offers